Goodbye Frizz, Hello Manageable ❧ Hair ❧

25 DIY Tea & Herbal Hair Rinse Recipes for Soft & Glowing Natural Hair

By B. CliShea

Goodbye Frizz, Hello Manageable Hair
25 DIY Tea & Herbal Hair Rinse Recipes
for Soft & Glowing Natural Hair
By B. **CliShea**

First Edition

https://www.clishea.co

Cover & Interior layout design by Mariana Vidakovics De Victor

Images from: https://pixabay.com/

Disclaimer
All information contained in this book is backed up by research and careful study. This book contains information about tea and herbal rinses, as well as recipes that you can try out yourself.
You can go ahead and try the rinses first in small amounts or in inconspicuous areas to ensure that you won't get any allergic reactions. If by any chance you feel any allergic reactions from using the recipes, feel free to visit a medical professional. Your safety should always be your top priority.

Welcome!

Welcome to **"Goodbye Frizz, Hello Manageable Hair: 25 DIY Tea & Herbal Hair Rinse Recipes for Soft & Glowing Natural Hair"**.

To thank you for your purchase, you're entitled to a special giveaway.[1]

---

1   https://www.instafreebie.com/free/xNCiP

Contents

Introduction

Thank you for grabbing a copy of this **Goodbye Frizz, Hello Manageable** Hair book!

Do you want to get rid of "bad hair days"?

Have you always experienced messy and tangled hair?

Do you always reach for a hat or any hair cover for that matter whenever someone takes your picture, lest be mocked?

Do you often struggle combing your hair, which makes you want to cut them all out?

If you answered 'yes' to any (or all) of those questions, then this book is for you. Don't worry; those moments will all come to an end, and will make sure that you have great hair, all day, every day.

This book is made to (hopefully) stop your "bad hair days", and make your everyday life feel like you've gone straight out of a shampoo commercial. Tangle-free hair, manageable strands... yes, they are possible through herbal and tea rinses.

Herbal and tea rinses are ideal if you wish to go natural for your hair. No unknown chemicals, no harmful ingredients. With herbal and tea rinses, you clearly know what's getting onto your head... literally.

Herbal and tea rinses are all filled with mild and safe ingredients – perhaps all of which can be found inside your kitchen cabinets. Making them is so easy too; the processes are almost the same for every recipe, all giving you glamorous hair.

Seems too good to be true? Maybe, but not really. There's one thing that's true, though - that you won't find out how it works until you try.

What are you waiting for? Flip the next page and start reading.

This book has seven chapters, each with its own discussion about herbal and tea rinses.

Here's a brief outline of this book:

Teas: Different Types, Different Kinds

This chapter is all about teas – what they are, and how they came about. This also discusses different tea varieties as well as the characteristics of each.

"What's the Right Herb for My Hair?"

For every hair type, there's a corresponding herb that will make it better. This chapter will teach you which herb will that be, and how you can use that herb for your hair. Whether your hair is dry, oily, or just normal with needs of its own, there will always be a right herb for your hair.

Basic Types of Hair Rinses

There are two basic types of hair rinses: the ACV or apple cider vinegar rinse, and the plain vinegar rinse. This chapter discusses both types as well as their similarities and differences. You can also find recipes for each type, should you want to concoct your own at the comfort of your home.

Herbal Rinses

This chapter *Herbal Rinses* will give you a brief background about them – definition, ingredients commonly used, and what good do you get out of using them. It will give you an idea why you should create the recipes you're about to find on the next chapter.

Herbal Rinse Recipes

After reading the goodness of herbal rinses, it's just understandable that you'd like to try them out yourself. Therefore, the next chapter will be filled with easy recipes for herbal rinses.

Tea Rinses

Tea rinses are quite similar to herbal rinses, but of course they're made with your favorite tea. In this chapter, you'll find what tea rinses are, what ingredients are commonly used, and what benefits do you get out of using them.

Tea Rinse Recipes

You can't leave tea rinses behind – there has to be a chapter for tea rinse recipes, don't you think? After learning what they can do for you, it's just right to create your own rinse and try them out yourself.

Where to Buy Herbs and Teas

No matter how hard you wish your hair to be better, you can't proceed to the next step if you don't have your ingredients on hand. In this chapter are suggested places and sites where you can buy your herbs and teas. Check them out and see why they are ideal places to grab your ingredients from.

Now that you have an idea of what the next chapters will bring you, it's now time to prepare yourself to learn more about herbs and teas, and to understand how to prepare herbal and tea rinse recipes.

Teas
Different Types, Different Kinds

Next to water, **tea** is the most consumed beverage in the world. It can be found on most US households – served hot, iced, flavored, on its own, anytime, anywhere.

This aromatic drink is prepared by pouring hot or boiling water over cured leaves of the *Camellia sinensis* plant.

Most of tea plants are grown in mountainous areas roughly 3,000 to 7,000 feet above sea level. They are grown in acidic and mineral-rich soil in between the Tropic of Cancer and Tropic of Capricorn. Biggest producers of tea include Argentina, Tanzania, China, Taiwan, India, Indonesia, Malawi, Kenya, Sri Lanka and Japan.

HOW TEA WAS DISCOVERED

Tea was discovered by a Chinese emperor named Shen-Nung. According to legends, there were tea leaves that accidentally got into the Emperor's pot of boiling water.

After originating in China where it was mainly consumed as a medicinal drink, soon, there were tea drinkers who drank it for recreation during the T'ang Dynasty. Tea drinking then spread to other East Asian countries.

It first came to Europe during the 16th century through Portuguese priests and merchants. Drinking tea then became a fashionable activity through the Britons in the 17th century, and had begun large-scale tea production and commercialization in India to stop the Chinese tea monopoly.

This drink has been present for more than 500 decades, and has evolved into a new element – the tea bag. Tea drinking, because of its benefits, is believed to stay for a long time.

DIFFERENT TYPES OF TEA

To those who aren't oriented with tea, there's more to tea than "hot" and "iced". There are various tea types to choose from. Each kind has its own aroma and taste, suited to fit the palates of tea drinkers worldwide.

Here's a guide to the different tea types:

Black Tea

This variant is the most common in the world. The leaves of the black tea are first allowed to wither completely before they undergo full oxidation. Referred to as "red tea" in China, younger black tea leaves are picked before they wither, and then rolled, oxidized and fired.

The oxidation results to the leaves' dark brown and black color, their more pronounced and robust flavors, and their higher caffeine content (when brewed appropriately).

The most well-known black teas come from various Indian regions such as Darjeeling, Assam and Nilgiri, and also come from Sri Lanka.

Recently, black tea leaves are processed by machines, but the black teas of best quality are those done by hand. Machine-processed black teas often end up with lower quality; these kinds are usually used in tea bags.

Green Tea

Green tea leaves are also allowed to wither but for much shorter time compared to black tea leaves. The leaves are heat-processed so they don't undergo oxidation – this results to the leaves retaining their color, plus achieving a more particular flavor with their accents and undertones. They are plucked, withered and then rolled.

They also end up having less caffeine compared to other tea variants.

The liquor's color don't often end up green, but rather, pale yellow. Green tea flavors usually range from toasty and grassy to fresh, steamed greens, or with mild and vegetable-like astringency.

Oolong Tea

Oolong (also spelled as "Wu Long") teas are semi-oxidized teas that have been grown in mainland China and Taiwan. Preparing oolong tea is time-consuming – perhaps the slowest – because it undergoes five steps, where rolling and oxidizing are performed repeatedly.

The caffeine content of oolong tea is somewhere between that of black tea and green tea. Its flavor may not be as robust as the black tea or as subtle as the green, but is more complex than those because of its own fragrant and mysterious tone. Their smooth yet rich flavors make them a top recommendation for those beginners to tea drinking.

Drinking oolong tea is often compared to eating fresh fruit or smelling fresh flowers because of their aromatic, fruity or even sweet tastes. Oolong tea is prepared by steeping them with hot but not boiling water for about 3 to 5 minutes. Oolong tea can be brewed multiple times.

White Tea

Compared to all other tea varieties, white tea undergoes the least processing. They're believed to be the most delicate out of all tea variants. Tea drinkers love how they have this subtlety yet so complex, and that they have this natural sweetness that can't be easily found in other tea types.

White tea doesn't undergo oxidation, and they are processed by hand through the tea plant's youngest shoots. It'll produce low amounts of caffeine if brewed in a low temperature and in a short steeping time.

White teas are steeped for about 2 to 3 minutes with water around 155 to 170 degrees. One tea serving can actually be brewed several times, with every steep revealing a new flavor.

Dark Tea

Dark tea is a probiotic tea that came from the Hunan and Sichuan provinces. This kind of tea is unique as it's the only kind that undergoes two fermentation processes. It's a good source of nutrients

The second fermentation process produces active microorganisms named Golden Flowers. You can actually see Golden Flowers in dark tea; those are the tiny yellow flecks on the tea itself.

It steeps up smoothly and gives a natural slightly sweet flavor.

Pu-erh Tea

This tea variety, the Pu-erh (or Puer) tea, is known as a subcategory of Dark Tea. This kind is post-fermented, which means its processing include not only fermentation but also prolonged storage under high humidity. It was named after a town in Yunnan Province, and true Pu-erh teas are believed to be valuable.

Puer teas are valued for their earthy taste and medicinal properties. This is a preferred drink by those who wish to lose weight, and has been recommended to those with high cholesterol because of its *lovastatin* content.

This tea variety has caffeine but not as high compared to other kinds, and so makes it an option for tea rinses. Still, it's believed to be the world's strongest tea. Puer can be prepared differently – it can be prepared bright, medium-bodied, or even slightly sweet.

BUYING TEA? HERE'S WHAT YOU SHOULD LOOK FOR

Unless you're from Asia, buying tea may end up being a tiring task. Sure, there's a lot of tea around, but how would you know which ones are actually the good ones?

If you want the good stuff, you have to really search for it. Of course, it'll always be recommended to buy the tea in person; you'll only know if you like it once you taste it. But since specialty teas are hard to find, then you'll have to rely on the Internet for that.

What should you look for when buying tea online? Take note of these guidelines.

Don't go straight to chains.

You know what they are – those found in large shopping districts and malls. These chains tend to carry those fancy ones more than pure straight tea variants – and the latter's what you want. Want lemongrass-lavender blends? Crave for chocolate chai tea? That's what they surely have, but if what you want is pure tea, then check other shops instead.

If you want quality tea, then look elsewhere. The teas they offer often have a lot of blends and additions that you no longer taste the actual tea. Their teas are bearable, but you can do better.

Think small.

You'd think that those stores that don't offer a lot of options are bad – their products may actually prove otherwise. Most good tea shops don't have large selections simply because what they offer are often handpicked by the owner, and specially chosen to fit one's taste.

Often, the owners of these small tea shops have visited tea farms – they visit mountains, talk to farmers, and taste tea themselves. After trying out different varieties, the owners go back to their shops with few kinds... carefully handpicked.

Compare that to shops that provide hundreds of tea types from different places around the world – do you think the owners would have the luxury of time to try them all out? Who knows, they might have, but it's highly possible they didn't and the teas all came from brokers.

That doesn't mean they're not offering quality tea, they possibly do. Still, the process of selection is still different; careful selections often produce quality results.

Ask questions if necessary.

Like with the other products, you don't often buy straight away at online stores – you browse products, compare them, and find out every little detail about them. There's a FAQ (frequently answered questions) page for that, but what if that page doesn't provide a response to your query?

If there's a phone number indicated for that store, then pick up the phone and give them a call. Employees should be more than happy to assist you and clarify whatever concerns you may have – there's nothing wrong with asking, especially if you're asking nicely. If tea fanatics are manning the store, then they'd love to discuss teas with you and share what you need to know.

Tea specialists exist.

Not every tea shop can provide all the answers to your questions and give you what you need. As previously discussed, tea shops often cater to a single (or maybe a few variants) tea type and may not have information about those that aren't in their stores.

If you're looking for a particular tea type, then go for those that have it as their specialty. Once you've found it, then you're lucky as they really know their stuff and even have diverse selections with regard to that tea type.

Quality Teas may cost more.

If you want good tea, then you have to be prepared to pay for it. It doesn't mean expensive tea is tea of high quality, though, and you don't have to crack the piggy bank open each time you wish to get your hands on good tea. You should be prepared, though, to pay more compared to prices you see on grocery stores.

Why does this happen? It's comparable to buying numerous servings of tea. A single serving corresponds to a few grams, and can even re-steeped. With this in mind, expensive teas can even cost just a dollar a cup.

Do you now have an idea on how you should buy your teas? Sounds time-consuming and mind-boggling, but once you've gotten the hang of it, you'd end up with best quality teas not only for drinking, but also for creating high-quality tea rinses.

"What's the Right Herb for My Hair?"

It's not enough that you know how to come up with herb and tea rinses; it's also important that you choose the best ingredients for your craft. To achieve shiny hair and nourished scalp, you have to pick the right components for your rinses.

Here are recommended herbs ideal for your hair rinses.

Lavender

Lavender can calm scalp inflammations and increase circulation to achieve better growth. It has antiseptic properties and its most popular use is as a treatment for dandruff or itchy scalp. Lavender is also believed to promote hair growth, not through an overnight treatment, but through regular massaging of the scalp.

Another known purpose of lavender is to relieve stress, and stress is one known cause of hair loss. Because lavender reduces stress and anxiety, it alleviates the chance of having hair loss and breakage.

Chamomile

Chamomile is an herb often used for hair treatments. Its special properties help prevent hair loss, and creating rinses with chamomile helps make hair stronger —

preventing tearing of hair and split ends. The antiseptic elements can remove dead cells and dirt that can obstruct hair follicles that stop hair from growing.

Chamomile can also soothe irritated scalp, and lead to prevention of dandruff. If you rinse with chamomile tea, you'll get nourished hair that has shine and glow. Plus, it can make hair brighter without having to damage it.

Calendula

Calendula helps soothe sensitive scalps and protect hair from free radicals. It also helps shield the scalp from bacterial growth. Herbal or tea rinse that includes calendula may add shine and even create warm highlights.

Calendula hydrates the scalp, and so it helps get rid of damaged scalp and dandruff. Because of this property, hair will grow stronger and help hair follicles grow better, leading to a thicker mane.

Hibiscus

Hibiscus flowers can do lots for your hair. Aside from treating scalp conditions such as hair loss and dandruff, it can also make your hair shiny and seal in moisture. Hair will also be tangle-free and get stronger as it grows longer.

Hibiscus can also bring red highlights to both light and dark hair. It is rich in vitamins A and C, as well as alpha hydroxyl acids and amino acids that all contribute to better hair conditions.

Basil not only feeds the scalp but also helps eliminate heavy metals and toxins from the body. The vitamins A and C in basil, as well as its flavonoids (orientin and vicenin) and polyphenolic acids help in promoting hair growth.

It also has lutein, zeaxanthin as well as essential oils such as citronellol, eugenol, terpineol, and limonene that provide its antibacterial and antiseptic properties. Basil also has vitamin K that helps with blood coagulation and bone strength.

Mint is known for its aroma and medicinal value. Mint helps you achieve shiny, soft and dandruff-free hair. It also stimulates your scalp as well as enhance hair growth. By improving the blood flow to the hair roots, hair becomes voluminous, and hair grows fuller and stronger.

Mint alone, or mint juice, can act as an aromatic hair conditioner. Applying this to your hair can make it smooth and frizz-free. Plus, it can revive and straighten hair if it has been worn out due to exposure to pollution and other harmful factors.

Nettle

Nettle is packed with vitamins and minerals. It has calcium, boron, magnesium, silica, and chromium, as well as vitamins A, B, C, D, and K. By stimulating the scalp, it improves blood circulation, resulting to a fuller and stronger hair. It also helps prevent loss and breakage of hair, and makes it soft and shiny.

Aside from improving hair's overall condition and appearance, it also can address different scalp issues such as dandruff and oily hair. Its antioxidative properties also directly affect one's skin and hair.

Horsetail

Horsetail has high silica amounts that help strengthen hair strands. The high concentrations of silicic acid can strengthen brittle, weak and damaged hair down to its core; it can even restore hair's body and luster. To add, horsetail can also treat oily scalps and help cure skin ailments such as eczema, psoriasis and dandruff.

You can find different minerals namely magnesium, calcium, chromium, potassium, iron, copper, bioflavonoids, etc. It's also good for oily hair because of its slight astringent properties. Just remember not to use a lot; because of its antiseptic properties, excessive amounts can end up drying your hair.

Rosemary

This herb encourages hair growth through improving the blood circulation to the scalp, made possible by the herb's component known as *ursolic acid*. Because of the ursolic acid in rosemary, more oxygen and nutrients will be brought to the hair follicles and then leads to healthy hair growth.

It also helps hair become strong and healthy, as well as increase its manageability and shine. Rosemary's revitalizing and stimulating properties help condition both hair and scalp. It has anti-inflammatory, antiseptic and antimicrobial effects. It's a remedy for itchiness, scalp irritation and dandruff.

Sage

Sage has antibacterial and astringent properties. It also has antioxidant properties, and can sooth dry and itchy scalp. Sage can fight dandruff and remove residue from hair and scalp. It can also cover gray hairs and darken hair.

To add, sage has anti-allergic, antibiotic, and antiseptic properties. It also has zinc, magnesium, and potassium, as well as vitamins A and C. Another good thing about sage is that it helps remove shampoo and conditioner build-up on your hair, making it shiny and soft.

Here's a quick summary of different herbs that will work best for your hair, as well as herbs that will help you in various hair and scalp conditions.

For Red Highlights	
Calendula	Henna
Red Clover flowers	Red Rose Petals
Hibiscus flowers	Rosehips

For Dark Highlights		
Black Tea	Comfrey Root	Sage
Nettle	Rosemary	Black Walnut Hulls

For Golden Highlights	
Sunflower petals	Chamomile
Lemon	Calendula

For Oily Hair and Scalp				
Bay leaf	Lavender	Chamomile	Peppermint	Rosemary
Thyme	Burdock root	Witch Hazel (bark)	Horsetail	Lemon Balm
Calendula	Lemongrass	Nettle	Lemon peel	Yarrow (both leaf and flower)

For Dry Scalp and Hair			
Burdock root	Marshmallow root	Comfrey leaf	Parsley leaf
Elder flowers	Calendula	Chamomile	Lavender
Horsetail	Nettle	Sage	Geranium

For Normal Hair			
Watercress	Chamomile	Sage	Linden flowers
Parsley leaf	Rosemary	Horsetail	Lavender
Basil	Calendula	Nettle	

For Thinning and Hair Loss			
Sage	Nettle	Basil	Rosemary

For Dandruff			
Lavender	Burdock Root	Eucalyptus	Clary Sage
Sage	Tea Tree	Nettle	Southernwood
Peppermint	Rosemary	Thyme	

As you can see, herbs don't have to be limited to a single function – sage, for example, can be used not only to help cure thinning and hair loss, but also to maintain normal hair, as well as give dark highlights.

Hair Rinses
Basic Types

There are two main types of hair rinses: apple cider rinse and vinegar rinse. How are these two defined and what are their differences from one another?

APPLE CIDER VINEGAR RINSE

An apple cider vinegar (ACV) rinse is a perfect inclusion to your hair care rituals. Various benefits of an ACV can include:

* *Increasing hair's shine.* Cuticles (the hair's outer layers) that are in good shape, unbroken and lying flat, will give hair a smooth appearance.
* *Stimulating the scalp.* Vinegar can promote blood circulation inside the small capillaries, and this action brings essential nutrients to the scalp, hence encouraging hair growth and making roots stronger.
* *Removes tangles and frizz.* ACV helps smoothen the cuticle, which leads to less tangles and frizz.
* *Decreases build-up.* An ACV rinse will remove residue and build-up on the hair shafts; this cleans the hair and scalp without having to strip the hair of its natural oils.
* *Adds volume to hair.* ACV doesn't weigh down hair strands with chemicals that cause hair to look limp and feel heavy. Because it removes build-up and frizz,

hair gets to have volume regardless of hair type, and naturally curly hair becomes bouncy.

* *Decreases dandruff and removes flakes.* Because of ACV's natural antifungal and antibacterial properties, it can help treat dry and itchy scalp. Without using harsh chemicals, fungus and bacteria associated with dandruff are killed and even help treat other scalp conditions.

How to Choose the Apple Cider Vinegar for Your Rinse

Finding a bottle of ACV is easy – there are different ACV brands out there to choose from. Picking out one that will give you the most health and beauty benefits is what's difficult.

Those ACV brands that appear clear and attractive may grab your attention faster, but since they're already pasteurized, the benefits may have already been lost. Go for those vinegars that appear cloudy and have sediments (also known as the "Mother") on the bottom part – that means they are organic and raw, and that they have all the enzymes and bacteria needed for its effectiveness.

Creating Your Own ACV Rinse

It's easy to come up with your own apple cider vinegar rinse.

Just take note of these steps and you'll soon have better hair, thanks to ACV:

* Mix a cup of water with 2 to 4 tablespoons of vinegar for your rinse.

* After shampooing and thoroughly rinsing your hair, pour the mixture slowly over your scalp. Allow it to flow down your hair's length; be careful to not let it get in your eyes.
* Massage the ACV mixture on your scalp; doing so will stimulate circulation as well as hair growth.
* Rinse out the vinegar after a minute or two.

You don't have to strictly follow the ratio mentioned; you can adjust the amount of vinegar according to your hair type. For those who have dry hair, you may want to start out with two tablespoons of vinegar. For those who have oily hair or dandruff, then it's better to start with three or four spoons of vinegar.

Feel free to adjust the blend depending on what works with your hair the most.

(WHITE) VINEGAR RINSE

Don't have apple cider vinegar around? Don't worry, plain white vinegar will also work just fine. Yes, white vinegar isn't just for cooking – it's also a good ingredient for hair rinses because of the benefits it brings, such as:

* *Cleanses and clarifies hair* – Using a lot of products for your hair may cause build-up and residue. Washing your hair with vinegar can remove this build-up and bring the shine back to your hair.
* *Balances the hair's natural pH levels* – Shampoos and other chemical-filled products strip the hair's natural protection and remove the natural oils secreted by the scalp that protects the hair from fungus and bacteria.

* *Reduces frizz* – Vinegar has soothing properties that smooth down hair cuticles, making your hair free from frizz for a long time.
* *Reduces hair's porosity* – Hair, when treated and exposed to different elements, can be damaged and lose its moisture. Once hair is damaged, it'll be hard to treat but you can use vinegar to protect new hair strands. How would you know your hair's porosity? Drop a strand in water: it sinks if it's porous and floats if it's not.
* *Prevents breakage and hair loss* – Vinegar makes hair smooth and tangle-free, hence combing your hair will be less difficult and lead to less breakage. This also leads to less split ends, which ends up with better hair.

How to Create Your Own Vinegar Rinse

Making your own vinegar rinse is very easy. Here's how:

* Mix a cup of water with 2 tablespoons of vinegar.
* Pour the mixture inside a squeeze bottle, and pour the liquid on your hair and scalp. Make sure the mixture won't get into your eyes.
* Rinse the mixture out with water after a few minutes.
* Use this mixture for about once or twice a week to achieve gorgeous hair.

White Or Acv?

If you wanted a natural vinegar rinse for your hair, then you have two choices: you can either go for apple cider vinegar or white vinegar.

What if you have both inside your pantry and you're finding it difficult to choose? How will you know which one suits you better?

One major factor to consider is if you're allergic to ACV or not. Not everyone can tolerate certain ingredients and can even be allergic to them. Apple cider vinegar, for example, may be a known component of various herbal recipes but not everyone can consume apple cider vinegar.

If you're allergic to ACV, then go for white vinegar instead. ACV may be preferred by more because they have slightly higher amounts of vitamins and minerals, but by using white vinegar, you'll still get the same benefits.

You also have to remember that white vinegar's pH levels are higher than that of ACV's. And so, if you choose to use white vinegar, then you should use more water to tone down the concentration. White vinegar can end up drying your hair if you don't use the right levels.

The smell of white vinegar is more intense compared to that of ACV's, but if you wish to use white vinegar, then you can add essential oils to remove the pungent smell, and/or add more water to dilute it further. You're still going to get soft and shiny hair by using this rinse.

HOW LONG RINSES LAST

Once you've determined which type of rinse works for your hair the best – whether it's an ACV rinse, herbal rinse, white vinegar rinse or tea rinse – you might want to consider making large batches to save time.

Because the hair rinses don't have preservatives, they will stay good when kept inside the refrigerator for maybe up a week. If they're still around, there might have molds and bacteria that has grown in it – sometimes visible, sometimes not.

If you went for making large batches, then one recommended way of storing them is to freeze them on ice trays. Depending on your hair's length, then you might be using about 2 to 3 cubes. Just leave the trays outside to unfreeze them; if you're in a hurry, then pour hot water.

Herbal Rinses

Homemade herbal rinses are full of antioxidants, minerals and nutrients that will help you take care of your hair.

Herbal rinses are recommended in place of store-bought conditioners because they don't have synthetic components such as various chemicals or preservatives found in some conditioners. Herbal rinses are completely pure and natural, plus they are quite simple to make.

There are three main reasons for using herbal rinses:

* For Hair Color and Enrichment
* To Add Nutrients and Vitamins to Hair and Scalp
* To Help Treat Hair and Scalp Conditions

BENEFITS OF HERBAL RINSES

People choose to go for herbal hair rinses because of the benefits they get out of it, namely:

* Protecting and enhancing hair color.
* Adding minerals and nutrients to hair and scalp, and
* Fighting hair and scalp issues.

Each benefit will be discussed in further detail, plus provide herbs that will help you achieve these benefits at maximum levels.

Hair Color Protection and Enhancement

Herbal rinses such as the burdock leaf tea can cleanse the system and can also give colored hair more shine inside and out. Herbal rinses can also add body and luster to hair.

Those with blonde hair can restore the hair's brightness through herbs and spices such as chamomile and calendula. Those with dark hair can also rely through herbs to make their hair even darker. Want gray hair to be darker? Herbs can also help you out with that.

Want to see which herb works best for your hair color? Check these out.

For Blonde Hair	
Chamomile	Sunflower Petals
Lemon Peel	Mullein Flowers
Calendula	Saffron
Marigold	Yarrow

For Red Hair	
Carrots	Hibiscus Flowers
Marigold	Red Rose Petals
Red Clover	Rosehips
Beets	Calendula

For Dark Brown Hair	
Rosemary	Sage
Cinnamon	Comfrey Root
Nettle	Cloves
Black Walnut Hulls	

For Dark Hair	
Marjoram	Rosemary
Blue Malva Flowers	Sage

Those herbs are often found in recipes to enhance or improve one's hair color. See which herbs correspond to your hair color the best.

Adds Minerals and Nutrients

Herbs contain minerals and other nutrients that benefit not only the skin and hair, but the whole body. The nutrients obtained from herbs make them capable of improving the state of hair, skin and body.

Examples of nutrient-packed herbs include nettles and alfalfa. Nettles, for one, contain minerals such as phosphorus, potassium, iron, cobalt, manganese, sodium, chromium, and selenium.

Combats Hair and Scalp Issues

Herbs are known to fight hair and scalp issues. Sage, for example, can fight baldness and hair loss because of its beta-sitosterol compound.

If you're dealing with hair loss or thinning, there's nettle, basil, sage and rosemary for you. For other scalp conditions, herbs such as yarrow, lavender and lemon will come to your rescue.

Herbal Rinse
Recipes

There are different kinds of herbal rinses depending on your needs. Do you need your hair color enhanced and enriched? What about acquiring the required nutrients and solving scalp conditions? There are herbal rinses for each.

FOR DRY HAIR

Licorice and Hibiscus Deep Conditioning Rinse

Because of the mucilage (a slippery substance) in the flowers and leaves of hibiscus, it's known as an excellent hair conditioner. It also helps soothe scalp irritation, reduce hair loss and lessen gray hair.

Licorice moisturizes the scalp and hair, plus has anti-inflammatory and antioxidant properties for stimulation of hair follicles and soothing irritated scalp.

Hibiscus can add a hint of red to the hair.

WHAT YOU NEED:
- Licorice, 1 stick or 1 tbsp. if powdered
- Hibiscus flowers, 1 to 2 if fresh, 1 tbsp. if dried
- Honey, 1 tsp.
- Water, 2 cups

PROCEDURE:

See last part for procedure.

Linden-Flower Hair Rinse

Sometimes hair gets dyed too often and become dry and brittle as a result. Linden-flower helps strengthen overly brittle hair as well as promote circulation -- new hair will then grow in healthier.

INGREDIENTS:
- Boiling water, 2 cups
- Linden-flowers, 2 tsp.

PROCEDURE:

Pour boiling water over the flowers; steep until cool. Strain the flowers and set the liquid aside.

HOW TO USE:

Wash your hair with shampoo, and thoroughly rinse with water. Pour the rinse over clean hair, and massage it onto scalp.

FOR OILY HAIR

Lemon is ideal for oily hair because of its tonic and astringent properties. It also soothes scalp irritation, dandruff and revitalizes hair and scalp. Mint, on the other hand, not only cools the hair and scalp but also increase the blood flow towards the scalp.

If used regularly, this lemon rinse can lighten the hair.

WHAT YOU NEED:
- Water, 2 cups
- Lemon or lime peel, 1 tsp.
- Mint leaves, 1 tbsp. if fresh or ½ tbsp. if dried

PROCEDURE:

This lavender and tea tree cleanser helps in cleaning the hair and fighting bacteria; it also gives off a fragrant scent. This is ideal for those who have dandruff, oily skin and are regular scalp infections.

INGREDIENTS:
- Distilled water, 4 cups
- Apple Cider Vinegar or white vinegar (whichever is available), ¼ cup
- Lavender, ¾ cup, dried
- Tea tree oil, 4 drops

PROCEDURE:

Combine all ingredients (except for the tea tree oil) in a pan. Place over low heat and let it boil. The buds should sink at the bottom after half an hour.

Remove the pan from the heat. Let it cool, and then add the tea tree oil.

HOW TO USE

You can use this rinse either with your regular shampoo or on its own. Just make sure to shake the bottle well, or else you won't get the actual mixture once the other components settle at the bottom of the bottle.

You can store this rinse inside the fridge, or even inside the shower. It will have a shorter shelf life during the summer, but will last longer during the winter.

Tea Tree and Lemon Scalp Rinse

Here's another rinse that uses lemon and tea tree. Remember to not use too much lemon – it may lighten your hair, but it can also end up drying your hair.

INGREDIENTS:
- Hot water, 3 cups
- Lemon juice, freshly squeezed, 4 tbsp.
- Tea tree oil, 5 drops

PROCEDURE:

Mix lemon juice and tea tree oil with hot water.

HOW TO USE:

Pour the mixture over your hair; make sure it won't get

into your eyes. Massage the mixture on your scalp and rinse thoroughly.

Mint and Rosemary Herbal Rinse

INGREDIENTS:

- Mint Leaves, 1 Tbsp.
- Rosemary Leaves, 1 Tbsp.
- Lemon, 1 Pc.
- Hot Water, 1 Cup

PROCEDURE:

Steep mint leaves, rosemary leaves and lemon juice in hot water for about 15 minutes. Strain the leaves afterwards and set the rinse aside.

HOW TO USE:

Shampoo your hair first; once done, use infusion as a final rinse.

Lavender Rinse

INGREDIENTS:

- Lavender flowers, 1 tbsp. fresh or ½ tbsp. dried
- Witch Hazel, 1 tsp. leaves/bark (optional)
- Water, 2 cups

PROCEDURE:

Combine lavender flowers with water inside a stainless-steel pan. Bring the mix to a boil. Reduce the flame; let it simmer for about 2 to 3 minutes. Switch off the heat, place the lid on the pot and let it steep until the pan cools. Strain the herbs once the pan has reached room temperature.

HOW TO USE:

Pour mixture over hair. Massage your scalp gently and allow your hair to use up all the rinse. There's no need to wash with water; it can serve as your final rinse.

FOR DAMAGED HAIR

Beer and Rosemary Herbal Infusion

INGREDIENTS:

- Rosemary, 1 tbsp.
- Hot water, 1 cup
- Beer, 2 tbsp.
- Juice of 1 Lemon

PROCEDURE:

Steep rosemary in hot water. Mix the lemon juice and beer afterwards. Wait for the rinse to reach room temperature; strain the herbs afterwards and set the liquid aside.

HOW TO USE:

Use mixture as a final rinse after washing your hair with shampoo.

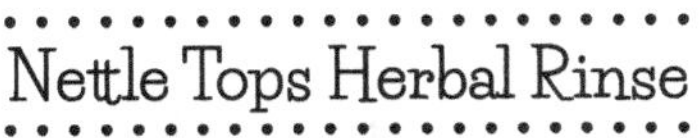

Nettle Tops Herbal Rinse

INGREDIENTS:

- Nettle tops. 2 ounces (Can use 2 Nettle tea bags or 4 tbsp. dried nettle)
- Water, 2 cups

PROCEDURE:

Add nettle tops to 2 cups of hot (almost boiling) water. Remove from heat and allow to steep for about 15 minutes. Strain the leaves and set aside.

HOW TO USE:

Apply hair rinse to clean both hair and scalp. Massage scalp gently; no need to rinse with water.

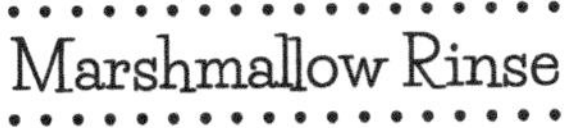

Marshmallow Rinse

INGREDIENTS:

- Water, 2 cups
- Marshmallow Root, 2 tbsp.
- Almond or argan oil (optional)

PROCEDURE:

Combine marshmallow root and water in a pan. Bring the mix to a boil. After a few minutes, reduce the flame. Let the mix simmer for about 2 to 3 minutes. Switch off the stove, cover the pot and let it steep until it reaches room temperature. After straining the herbs, it will then be ready to use.

After washing your hair with your regular shampoo, pour the mixture over hair. Gently massage your scalp and soak your hair in the rinse for about 5 minutes. Rinse hair using clean water, and allow your hair to dry naturally.

FOR ALL TYPES OF HAIR

Rosemary-Thyme Rinse

Both herbs, rosemary and thyme, have antiseptic properties that help scalp clean and healthy. They are also known to keep hair soft and silky. You'll notice your hair darken subtly and naturally after several rinses.

Ingredients:
- Rosemary leaves, 1 tbsp. if fresh and ½ tbsp. if dried
- Thyme leaves, 1 tbsp. if fresh, and ½ tbsp. if dried
- Boiling water, 2 cups

Procedure:
- Combine herbs in a glass bowl; pour boiling water afterwards.
- Let leaves steep and wait until cool.
- Strain liquid and transfer into a clean container.

How to Use:
After washing your hair with shampoo, use the mixture as a final rinse. Do not rinse with water.

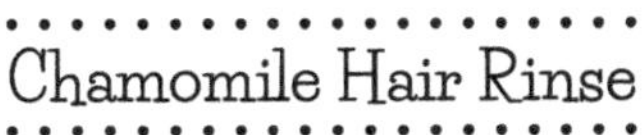

Chamomile Hair Rinse

INGREDIENTS:
- Filtered water, ½ cup
- Apple cider vinegar, ½ cup
- Chamomile flowers, 2 tbsp.

PROCEDURE:
- Boil chamomile flowers and water for about 15 minutes.
- Wait for the mixture to cool, and then strain the flowers afterwards.
- Mix in the vinegar.

HOW TO USE:
You can either use the mixture as a final rinse, or just simply pour over your head in the shower.

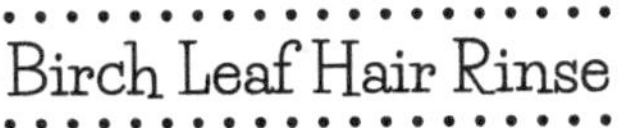

Birch Leaf Hair Rinse

This rinse can help prevent hair loss and keep your hair and scalp healthy if used regularly. It can also make the hair softer, shinier and darker over time.

INGREDIENTS:
- Boiling Water, 2 cups
- Birch Leaves, dried, 2 tsp.

PROCEDURE:
Steep birch leaves in boiling water for a few minutes until cool. Strain the leaves and set the mixture aside.

Pour the mixture over clean hair. Massage into scalp. You can choose to leave it on hair or to rinse after a few minutes.

If you're allergic to celery, wild carrots, mug wort and certain spices, then check first with your physician before trying out this hair rinse.

Elderberry Mix

Ingredients:
- Fresh Elderberries, 1 cup
- Water, 1 pint
- Vinegar, 1 tbsp.

Procedure:

Simmer fresh elderberries in water for about 15 to 20 minutes. Strain elderberries and set aside.

To prepare vinegar water, mix a tablespoon of vinegar to a cup of water.

How to Use:

Apply elderberry rinse to hair and wait for 15 minutes. Rinse hair using vinegar water.

Tea Rinses

Teas are made not only for drinking, but also for improving health and wellness, such as that of your hair.

Tea rinses are effective because of their caffeine content, which penetrates the hair follicles and give the hair the boost that they need. It may stimulate hair growth; however, no guaranteed length can be stated.

Perform tea rinses properly and in moderation; small caffeine amounts may increase hair growth, but too much caffeine can bring the opposite and stop hair growth as a response.

Among the different varieties of tea, black tea is least recommended because of its high caffeine content. If your only available option is black tea, then make sure to dilute it to weaken the tea's strength.

Other tea varieties are good to be used in tea rinses, and every tea type has its corresponding hair type or condition.

BENEFITS OF TEA RINSES

What do you get out of washing your hair with tea? Here are the benefits you get from tea rinses:

* Increased Hair Growth
* Less Hair Shedding
* Restores or Brightens Your Hair Color
* Prevents Hair Breakage

The benefits you get from tea mostly come from the tea's caffeine. Because of the tea's caffeine content, teas can affect the hair and make it better.

Increased Hair Growth

From green tea, you'll get polyphenols, Vitamin C and Vitamin E – vitamins that help stimulate hair growth and make hair softer. That's why green tea is also a main component for shampoos and conditioners – it helps make hair shinier and more lustrous.

Green tea also helps prevent hair loss because of its anti-inflammatory properties, plus due to its polyphenolic substances that are stress-inhibitory. People lose hair because of stress; by drinking tea, they avoid stress brought by its relaxing effect.

Less Hair Shedding

By inhibiting dihydrotestosterone (DHT) that stops hair growth and causes hair fall, tea helps stimulate hair growth. The components of tea can react with the body's testosterone; tea influences their levels and balance their amounts in the blood so it won't become DHT and lead to hair loss.

Tea can also help treat dandruff through its antiseptic properties. Tea reduces inflammation, and so it prevents and even cures psoriasis and dandruff. Further, tea can exfoliate dry flakes that had formed on the scalp due to dandruff.

Prevents Hair Breakage

Because of the components found in tea, hair becomes stronger as it gets longer. It helps prevent hair breakage by protecting each strand, and stronger hair also means less split ends.

Tea can also achieve hair regrowth and reduce patterns of hair loss because of its catechin component. Aside from stimulating hair growth, it also aids cardiovascular activity as well as micro capillary blood circulation towards the hair follicles.

Tea Rinse
Recipes

Want to try out tea rinse recipes for your hair? Check out these recipes and see which ones will work for your hair the best.

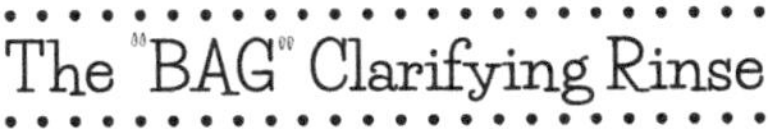

The "BAG" Clarifying Rinse

In this clarifying rinse, "BAG" stands for beer, ACV and green tea, its main ingredients. Beer can bring shine, body and luster to your hair, so it'll work well with ACV and green tea for your strands.

INGREDIENTS:
- Water, 6 cups
- Peppermint, Eucalyptus or Tea Tree Oil (whichever you prefer), 3-6 drops
- Any light beer *(flat)*, 1 small can
- Green tea, 2-3 bags
- Apple Cider Vinegar, ¼ cup

PROCEDURE:
- * Steep the green tea bags on boiling water.
- * Have a large glass bowl and place water with green tea, essential oils, ACV and beer. Wait until cool to touch.

HOW TO USE:
This mixture can either be used in place of shampoo,

or as a final rinse after washing the hair. Pour over hair, massage onto scalp and hair for about 2-3 minutes. Rinse afterwards with lukewarm water. Repeat if needed.

Green Tea Hair Rinse

INGREDIENTS:
- Green Tea, 2 Tea Bags
- Boiling Water, 2 Cups
- Honey, 1 Tbsp. (Optional)

PROCEDURE:

Prepare a strong cup of green tea by brewing 2 green tea bags and water. Let tea cool down to lukewarm prior to using. You can add a tablespoon of honey for more softness and shine to your hair.

HOW TO USE:

Clean your hair using shampoo and/or conditioner. Let hair stay damp. Spray or pour tea slowly onto the scalp and massage through hair. Leave tea on hair for about 30 minutes; wear a shower or plastic cap if preferred. Rinse mix with cold water.

INGREDIENTS:

- Black tea, 3 to 4 tea bags
- Boiling Water, 2 cups

PROCEDURE:

Prepare strong black tea by brewing 3 to 4 tea bags with 2 cups of boiling water. Allow the tea to cool down before using it on your hair.

HOW TO USE:

Cleanse hair with shampoo and/or conditioner. Pour tea on scalp and massage thoroughly. Leave black tea on scalp and hair for about 45 minutes, and then rinse with cold water.

Raspberry Leaf, Sage, Rosemary and Walnut Hulls Tea

INGREDIENTS:

- Black Walnut Hulls, chopped or in powder form, 2 g
- Rosemary, 2 grams
- Red Raspberry Leaf, 2 grams
- Sage, 2 grams
- Black Tea

PROCEDURE:

Brew black tea; add all other ingredients (red raspberry leaf, rosemary, sage and black walnut hulls) afterwards. Let ingredients steep for a while and wait until mixture has reached room temperature.

After the mixture has cooled down, strain it. Add more water to make it a quart.

How to Use:

Wash your hair with shampoo and conditioner as normal. Rinse hair thoroughly with water. Pour the black tea mixture slowly through hair and massage scalp afterwards. No need to rinse with water.

Rooibos Tea for Red Hair

Ingredients:
- Hibiscus Flowers, 4 grams
- Red Clover, 2 grams
- Calendula, 2 grams
- Rooibos Tea, 2 oz.

Procedure:

Brew rooibos tea; add calendula, hibiscus flowers and red clover afterwards. Wait until brewed tea reaches room temperature before using. Add water to make it reach at least a quart of liquid.

How to Use:

Wash and rinse your hair as normal. Pour mixture afterwards on hair and scalp; massage scalp thoroughly. Let tea stay on hair and scalp; no need to rinse with water.

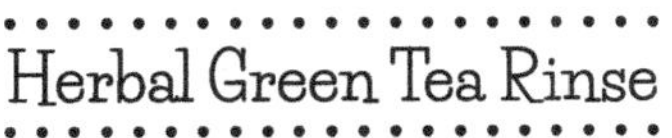

Herbal Green Tea Rinse

INGREDIENTS:

- Green Tea
- Comfrey Leaves, 2 grams
- Burdock Root, 2 grams
- Nettle, 2 grams
- Calendula, 2 grams

PROCEDURE:

Prepare green tea with the rest of the ingredients. Let ingredients steep for about 2 minutes and wait until tea reaches room temperature. After the tea has cooled down, strain other ingredients and set tea aside.

HOW TO USE:

Cleanse your hair as normal. Pour the mixture on hair and scalp. No need to rinse with water.

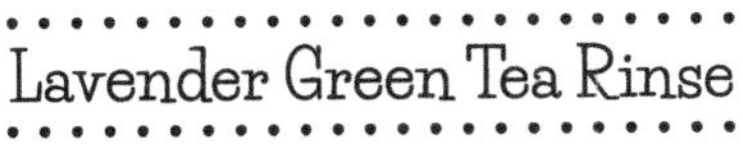

Lavender Green Tea Rinse

INGREDIENTS:

- Green Tea
- Lavender, 2 grams

PROCEDURE:

Mix lavender and green tea in a pan. Bring the mix to a boil. Lower the heat and allow the mixture to simmer for about 2 to 3 minutes. Turn off the heat and let it steep until it reaches room temperature. Strain the herbs out and use as normal.

How to Use:

You can choose to use the rinse as a substitute to shampoo, or as a final rinse after you've washed your hair with shampoo and/or conditioner.

Green Tea Rinse

Ingredients:

- Green Tea, 2 bags
- Hot Water, 2 to 3 cups

Procedure:

Steep green tea bags in hot water. Wait until the tea reaches room temperature before you can use it on your hair and scalp.

How to Use:

This green tea rinse can be used as a final rinse for your hair; massage the rinse on your scalp for about a minute or two.

Black Tea Rinse

Ingredients:

- Black tea, 2 to 4 bags
- Water, 2 cups

PROCEDURE:

Add 2 to 4 black tea bags to boiled water. Allow it to steep for a few hours or until the tea has reached room temperature. Remove the tea bags and set liquid aside.

HOW TO USE:

Pour the tea rinse on your hair and scalp after shampooing. Let sit for 20 to 30 minutes. For best results, deep condition your hair after doing the tea rinse.

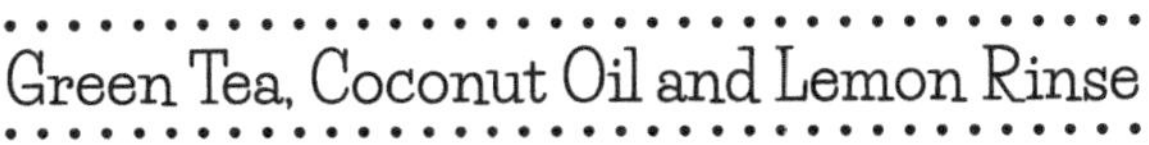

Green Tea, Coconut Oil and Lemon Rinse

INGREDIENTS:

- Green tea leaves, 2 tbsp.
- Coconut oil, 1 tbsp.
- Lemon peel, 1 pc.
- Water, 1 cup

PROCEDURE:

Boil a cup of water and then add the green tea leaves. Add the coconut oil and lemon peel as well. Heat for 2 minutes, and then allow it to cool completely.

HOW TO USE:

Apply this mixture on hair and scalp using a cotton ball. Massage the mixture on your scalp for a few minutes. After 45 minutes, rinse it off with shampoo.

WHERE TO BUY
Herbs and Teas

The quality of the herbal and tea rinses you're making will largely depend on the ingredients you use to come up with the mixture. No matter how well you steep the herbs or how you prepare the teas, it won't be as effective if your ingredients aren't at their best.

How would you know if the tea or herb you're using is ideal for a hair rinse? Where should you buy them to be assured that you're getting the best quality?

The answers will be found in this chapter.

WHICH IS BETTER – ONLINE STORES OR GROCERY STORES?

Basically, there are two ways on how you can have herbs and teas on hand: order herbs online, or purchase them on supermarkets and grocery stores.

Which option is better?

Each option would have its own advantages and disadvantages; see which one suits your needs better.

Grocery Stores. The grocery store's number one offering is convenience. After paying for the herb or tea, then it's yours to take home whether to add into your recipes or to mix in your organic rinses. You can go ahead and clean your hair with whatever concoction you wish to come up with.

Here's the "bad" part: their prices are way higher compared to online stores. Research actually shows that groceries' prices can be 3 to 20 times higher, so you might as well buy online – you'll probably get it cheaper even with shipping.

Online Stores. With the previous statements in mind, prices of herbs and teas on online stores are significantly cheaper. Sage, for example, can be bought online for about 76 cents, but can be bought at the grocery store for $16 an ounce.

What's the drawback with online stores? With online stores, you'd still have to wait before you can have the ingredients on hand. If you're lucky, you'd get it in a day or two, but for some, the waiting can last a week.

Plus, to grab the best deals, you might have to buy in bulk to make the most of the shipping fees. That means you'd end up with lots of herbs that will last you a few weeks or so.

So what's the verdict? If you need the herbs at this very minute and if you don't need a lot, then it might not hurt to buy at grocery stores for now. But if you see yourself using these herbs for a long time and that you're going to need a lot, then buy at online stores instead – a few days won't hurt if it means you'd have more herbs to use for your rinses.

RECOMMENDED ONLINE STORES: HERB EDITION

There are a lot of stores selling herbs and teas online. It's close to impossible to mention them all, but here are some of them that's highly recommended.

First stop: herbs.

Companion Plants (*companionplants.com*)

This is a site for an herb nursery established since 1982. They offer around 600 kinds of both common and exotic herb varieties, and they provide herbs of different purposes – medicinal, culinary, cosmetic, etc. Selections are sorted to make shopping easy and pleasurable for you.

If you wish to see their plants yourself, you can check out their physical store – actually their greenhouse – at Athens, OH wherein you can see these herbs for yourself. They ship anywhere in the country and make sure that your plants arrive at your doorstep safe and sound.

Mountain Valley Growers (*mountainvalleygrowers.com*)

Mountain Valley Growers started with 7 varieties in 1983, and grew to supplying around 400 varieties in 2002. This company is certified organic by the USDA, and aside from herbs, they also sell vegetable plants and flowers.

Aside from offering plants, they also help plant shoppers by including botanical name cross-referencing, plus have herb quick reference pages. By doing so, you'll be sure that you're buying what you really need. They also have social media pages to ensure they'll always be in touch with potential and existing customers.

Strictly Medicinal Seeds (*strictlymedicinalseeds.com*)

Strictly Medicinal Seeds has a wide variety of plants

for you. Their name might have 'seeds' on it, but don't be fooled – they have not only seeds, but plants of different shapes and sizes. They have herbs and extracts, live roots, trees and shrubs.

That's not all; they also have books and DVDs sold here if you need more education or if you wish to grow these plants yourselves. On that note, they also offer screens and other gardening supplies.

Richters (*richters.com*)

This site also offers a huge herb selection – they offer every type of herb plus their different varieties. A catalog is found on the site and is updated annually; you can check the catalog for the list of herbs they offer and see those ones available for pre-order or those on-hand. This helps you make an informed decision whenever you buy from them.

Richters hopes to help not only those casual buyers, but also those who rely on herbs for a living e.g. those who make herbal products or those in the herb business. They also have a gift shop and greenhouses located in Toronto; you can also check those out if you happen to be in the area.

RECOMMENDED ONLINE STORES: TEA EDITION

As previously discussed, finding quality tea could be difficult in a sense that you can't initially taste what you're paying for, unless you've already tried it out before.

To make online tea shopping easier, here are some of the quality tea stores.

Teavivre (*teavivre.com*)

This online tea store's specialty is Chinese tea. They only carry Chinese tea inside their store, but the ones they have are of good quality and quite incomparable. They also offer different kinds of pu-erh teas and often provide sales and discounts, which is good for those who are just beginners to this tea variety.

Their website may be quite simple, but you'll see how their simplicity gets the job done. The teas are grouped according to their types so you won't be lost in searching for what you need. You can also find tea sets and accessories to complete your tea experience.

Rishi (*rishi-tea.com*)

Rishi offers a wide variety of tea types; they're sure to provide the kind of tea you require. Aside from selling straight tea, Rishi also has teabags and blends. They may look like a big shop, but their tea offerings are of good quality.

There are Rishi teas that can be found on supermarkets, so you can try one out first and see the quality for yourself. Their teas have the USDA Organic logo and are free of genetically modified organisms (GMOs). To add, Rishi Tea products don't have ingredients that have dairy or gluten, and even follow strict control procedures for allergens.

Red Blossom Tea (*redblossomtea.com*)

The teas from the Red Blossom Tea Company are sourced from different growers and artisans in China and Taiwan. They conduct annual buying trips that happen the same as the Spring tea harvest.

The company admits that it could have been easier to buy through distributors or large markets but they believe that the effort they spend will lead to high quality teas as well as teawares. After 30 years of carefully selecting their tea, they have set high expectations within themselves and hope to always provide flavorful products.

Fang Gourmet Tea (*fangtea.com*)

This New York tea shop is said to offer one of the finest tea-tasting experiences in the area – they focus on blacks, Pu-erh and oolong teas from Taiwan and China. Their website may not be as updated, but customers can always talk to the company staff over the phone to ask what kind of teas they have on stock.

Aside from offering quality tea, they also have tea accessories to give you the complete tea-drinking experience. Want to try something new? They have pomelo tea, a rare specialty made when a pomelo is hollowed out, stuffed with tea leaves and aged prior to brewing.

In Pursuit of Tea (*inpursuitoftea.com*)

This company is one of those that has a wide range of tea varieties but does not compromise quality. It has been around since 2001, and their tea offerings have spanned from Himalayan to Japanese, to Chinese tea that have focused on Pu-erh and oolong teas.

In Pursuit of Tea believes that they should offer teas with natural aromas and flavors. The company looks for "true teas" and ensures they won't be mixed with ingredients of inferior quality. Their teas are not blended, that's why they maintain their complexity and diversity.

Everlasting Teas *(everlastingteas.com)*

The company was established in 2011 with the intent of bringing you loose leaf tea from Taiwanese farms. They don't just import tea – they go straight to specific individuals who have raised tea for generations.

Everlasting Tea has four main tea types: green, white, black and oolong. Their shop does not only have aged tea, but they also have younger teas that are also worth trying.

Crimson Lotus Tea *(crimsonlotustea.com)*

Crimson Lotus Tea specializes in pu-erh tea, as well as tea wares and tea education. Their teas come from Yunnan, while their company is based in Seattle. The company is owned by a couple who never thought they'll be in the tea business (the owner was first a coffee lover) but now is so obsessed about it.

The company is mainly about one-of-a-kind pu-erh teas, and they aim to attract the new tea drinkers. Every year, they go to Yunnan, China to be as close to their tea source as they can.

Whether you'll choose to buy your herbs and teas online or at a physical store will be solely up to you – go for whichever is more suitable for your needs. What's important is to have the herbs and teas that you need for your herbal and tea rinses.

Conclusion

Thank you for taking the time to read this book *"Homemade Tea & Herbal Rinses: 25 Easy DIY Recipes to Soften, Add Luster, and Create Manageability to Your Natural Hair"*.

Herbs and teas do not exist just for medicinal purposes, and they aren't around just for drinking. Herbs and teas are around because you can use them for aesthetic purposes, particularly for making your hair fuller and more beautiful.

After reading this book, you should then be more familiar with herbs and teas, their different types and their benefits. You should have learned as well how to make use of different herbs and teas to make your hair better.

Your next step is to try out the recipes listed in this book. We will expect you to have hair worthy of a shampoo commercial, won't we?

Again, thank you for grabbing a copy of this book. Hope you enjoyed it!